GUIDE TO SIMVASTATIN ZOCOR USAGE

A Quick and Easy Guide to Treat Heart Disease, Prevent Heart Attack and Strokes and Reduce High Cholesterol and Lipids.

Alexander Falleni

Disclaimer

The data gave on this stage is to instructive and educational purposes as it were. It isn't expected as a substitute for proficient clinical counsel, conclusion, or treatment. Continuously look for the counsel of your doctor or other qualified wellbeing supplier with any inquiries you might have in regards to an ailment. Never ignore proficient clinical guidance or postpone in looking for it in light of something you have perused on this stage.

Contents

CHAPTER ONE

Introduction to Simvastatin

What is Simvastatin?

Simvastatin is a medication belonging to the statin class, which is primarily used to lower cholesterol levels in the blood. By inhibiting the enzyme HMG-CoA reductase, Simvastatin effectively reduces the production of cholesterol in the liver. This action leads to lower levels of low-density lipoprotein (LDL) cholesterol, often referred to as "bad" cholesterol, while also increasing levels of high-density lipoprotein (HDL) cholesterol, known as "good" cholesterol.

History of Simvastatin Development

Simvastatin was first approved by the U.S. Food and Drug Administration (FDA) in 1991. It was developed from a natural product found in a fungus called Aspergillus, and its introduction marked a significant advancement in cardiovascular medicine. Over the years, extensive clinical research has established Simvastatin's efficacy in reducing cardiovascular events, making it one of the most widely prescribed medications for managing hyperlipidemia.

Importance in Cardiovascular Health

Given the high prevalence of cardiovascular diseases globally, Simvastatin plays a critical role in public health. Elevated cholesterol levels are a major risk factor for conditions such as heart attacks and strokes. By effectively managing these levels, Simvastatin contributes significantly to the prevention of such events and promotes overall heart health.

Current Use and Prescribing Trends

Today, Simvastatin is frequently prescribed not only for patients with high cholesterol but also for those at risk of cardiovascular diseases. Its ease of use, combined with favorable outcomes in clinical trials, has solidified its position in treatment guidelines. As research continues to evolve, healthcare providers are exploring new applications and benefits of this medication, ensuring that patients receive optimal care.

In summary, Simvastatin is a vital tool in the fight against cardiovascular disease, and understanding its role, mechanism, and applications is essential for both healthcare professionals and patients.

CHAPTER TWO

Indications and Uses

Primary Uses of Simvastatin

Simvastatin is primarily indicated for the following conditions:

Hyperlipidemia:

- Simvastatin is used to treat elevated levels of total cholesterol, LDL cholesterol, and triglycerides in patients diagnosed with hyperlipidemia. It helps lower these lipid levels, reducing the risk of cardiovascular events.

Prevention of Cardiovascular Disease:

- For individuals with existing cardiovascular conditions (such as coronary artery disease) or those at high risk (due to factors like diabetes, hypertension, or a family history of heart disease), Simvastatin is prescribed to prevent heart attacks, strokes, and other cardiovascular events.

Familial Hypercholesterolemia:

- In patients with familial hypercholesterolemia, a genetic disorder leading to extremely high cholesterol levels, Simvastatin is used to help manage cholesterol levels and reduce cardiovascular risk.

Off-Label Uses

While the primary indications are well-established, Simvastatin may also be prescribed for several off-label uses:

Post-Myocardial Infarction:

- o Some clinicians prescribe Simvastatin to patients recovering from a heart attack to help lower cholesterol and reduce the risk of future cardiovascular events.

Alzheimer's Disease:

- o Research has explored the potential neuroprotective effects of statins, including Simvastatin, in Alzheimer's disease. However, results are mixed, and this use is still under investigation.

Polycystic Ovary Syndrome (PCOS):

- o There is emerging interest in using Simvastatin for managing metabolic issues associated with PCOS, particularly for patients with elevated androgen levels and insulin resistance.

Combination Therapy

Simvastatin is often used in combination with other medications to enhance its lipid-lowering effects. For instance:

- **Ezetimibe**: This medication, which reduces intestinal absorption of cholesterol, can be combined with Simvastatin for a more comprehensive approach to managing cholesterol levels.
- **Niacin and Fibrates**: In certain cases, healthcare providers may recommend these agents alongside Simvastatin to further improve lipid profiles.

Guidelines for Use

Healthcare providers typically follow established guidelines for initiating and adjusting Simvastatin therapy based on individual patient profiles, including:

- Baseline lipid levels
- Cardiovascular risk factors
- Response to treatment
- Tolerance of the medication

Overall, Simvastatin's indications and uses highlight its importance in both managing lipid levels and preventing cardiovascular diseases, making it a cornerstone of cholesterol management in clinical practice.

CHAPTER THREE

Side Effects and Risks

Common Side Effects

While Simvastatin is generally well-tolerated, some patients may experience side effects. Commonly reported side effects include:

Muscle Pain and Weakness:

- o Myalgia (muscle pain) is one of the most frequently reported side effects. Some individuals may also experience muscle weakness (myopathy).

Gastrointestinal Issues:

- o Patients may experience nausea, diarrhea, constipation, or abdominal pain.

Headaches:

- o Some individuals report experiencing headaches while on Simvastatin.

Elevated Liver Enzymes:

- o In some cases, liver enzymes may become elevated, indicating potential liver issues. Regular monitoring of liver function tests is recommended.

Serious Risks

While serious side effects are less common, they can occur and require immediate medical attention:

Rhabdomyolysis:

- o A rare but severe condition characterized by the breakdown of muscle tissue, leading to the release of myoglobin into the bloodstream. This can result in kidney damage and is considered a medical emergency.

2. **Liver Damage**:
   o Although rare, significant liver damage can occur. Symptoms may include jaundice (yellowing of the skin or eyes), dark urine, and severe fatigue.

3. **Allergic Reactions**:
   o Some individuals may experience allergic reactions, including rash, itching, swelling, or difficulty breathing.

4. **Cognitive Effects**:
   o Some patients report memory loss or confusion while taking statins, though evidence is mixed and further research is needed.

Drug Interactions

Simvastatin can interact with several medications, potentially increasing the risk of side effects or reducing efficacy:

1. **Certain Antibiotics and Antifungals**:
    o   Medications such as erythromycin and ketoconazole can increase Simvastatin levels in the body, raising the risk of muscle-related side effects.
2. **Other Lipid-Lowering Agents**:
    o   Combining Simvastatin with other lipid-lowering medications, such as fibrates (e.g., gemfibrozil), may significantly increase the risk of muscle damage.
3. **Calcium Channel Blockers**:
    o   Certain medications like diltiazem can also elevate Simvastatin levels.

Monitoring and Management

To minimize risks, healthcare providers often recommend:

- **Regular Monitoring**: Routine blood tests to check liver function and lipid levels.
- **Patient Education**: Informing patients about potential side effects and signs of serious reactions.
- **Dosage Adjustments**: Modifying the dose based on individual response and tolerance.

In conclusion, while Simvastatin is effective for managing cholesterol levels, it is crucial for patients and healthcare providers to be aware of potential side effects and risks, ensuring that treatment remain safe and effective. Regular communication and monitoring are key to managing any adverse effects that may arise.

CHAPTER FOUR

Drug Interactions with Simvastatin

Simvastatin can interact with a variety of medications and substances, potentially increasing the risk of side effects or diminishing the effectiveness of treatment. Understanding these interactions is crucial for safe and effective therapy.

Major Drug Interactions

Fibrates:

- o **Gemfibrozil**: This medication significantly increases the risk of myopathy and rhabdomyolysis when combined with Simvastatin. If a fibrate is needed, fenofibrate is often preferred due to a lower interaction risk.

Antibiotics:

- o **Erythromycin** and **Clarithromycin**: These macrolide antibiotics can increase Simvastatin levels, heightening the risk of muscle-related side effects.

Antifungals:

- o **Ketoconazole** and **Itraconazole**: These medications can inhibit the metabolism of Simvastatin, leading to elevated blood levels and increased side effects.

Calcium Channel Blockers:

- o **Diltiazem** and **Verapamil**: These can increase Simvastatin levels, raising the risk of adverse effects. Dosage adjustments may be necessary.

HIV Protease Inhibitors:

- o **Ritonavir**: This medication can significantly elevate Simvastatin levels, which may lead to severe muscle issues.

Other Statins:

- o Combining Simvastatin with other statins is generally not recommended due to an increased risk of adverse effects.

Other Notable Interactions

Grapefruit Juice:

- o Grapefruit and its juice can inhibit the enzyme CYP3A4, which is involved in the metabolism of Simvastatin. This can lead to higher blood levels of the drug and increase the risk of muscle-related side effects.

Certain Antidepressants:

- **Fluoxetine** and **Sertraline**: These medications may interact with Simvastatin, necessitating careful monitoring.

Immunosuppressants:

- **Cyclosporine**: Co-administration can significantly raise Simvastatin levels and increase the risk of serious side effects.

Recommendations for Management

- **Review Medication History**: Healthcare providers should conduct a thorough review of all medications a patient is taking, including over-the-counter drugs and supplements.

- **Monitor for Side Effects**: Patients should be informed about the signs of potential side effects, particularly muscle pain or weakness.

- **Consider Alternative Therapies**: If significant interactions are identified, alternative therapies or adjusted dosages may be necessary to ensure patient safety.

Being aware of potential drug interactions with Simvastatin is essential for optimizing treatment and minimizing risks. Regular communication between patients and healthcare providers can help manage these interactions effectively, ensuring the best possible outcomes in cholesterol management.

CHAPTER FIVE

Dosage and Administration

Recommended Dosages

The dosage of Simvastatin is individualized based on the patient's condition, cholesterol levels, and response to treatment. The following guidelines provide a general framework for prescribing:

Initial Dosage:

- **Adults**: The typical starting dose is **10 to 20 mg** once daily in the evening.
- **Higher Risk Patients**: For individuals with significantly elevated cholesterol levels or those at higher risk for cardiovascular events, a starting dose of **40 mg** may be considered.

Maintenance Dosage:

- **Usual Range**: The maintenance dose can range from **10 mg to 40 mg** once daily, depending on the individual's lipid profile and tolerance.
- **Maximum Dose**: The maximum recommended dose is **40 mg** per day. In some specific cases, such as those on other cholesterol-lowering medications, a dose of **80 mg** may be used, but this is typically reserved for patients already stabilized on this dose and closely monitored for side effects.

Administration Guidelines

- **Timing**: Simvastatin should be taken once daily in the evening. Cholesterol synthesis is highest during the night, so evening dosing enhances its effectiveness.

- **With or Without Food**: Simvastatin can be taken with or without food, but consistent timing helps with adherence.

Special Populations

Elderly:

- Dosing should be cautious and individualized, often starting at the lower end of the dosage range (e.g., 10 mg).

Patients with Renal Impairment:

- Dosage adjustments may be necessary for patients with significant renal impairment. Generally, starting at a lower dose is recommended, with careful monitoring.

Patients with Liver Disease:

- Simvastatin is contraindicated in patients with active liver disease. For those with mild to moderate liver impairment, careful monitoring is essential, and dose adjustments may be required.

Pediatric Use

- Simvastatin is approved for use in children aged **10 years and older** for familial hypercholesterolemia. The recommended starting dose is **10 mg**, with a maximum dose of **40 mg**. Close monitoring of lipid levels and side effects is crucial.

Monitoring and Follow-Up

- **Lipid Levels**: Lipid levels should be checked within **4 to 12 weeks** after initiating or adjusting the dose of Simvastatin. Subsequent monitoring can be done every 3 to 12 months, depending on the patient's condition.

- **Liver Function Tests**: Baseline liver function tests should be conducted before starting treatment, with follow-up tests as clinically indicated, especially if there are signs of liver issues.

Proper dosing and administration of Simvastatin are critical for achieving desired lipid-lowering effects while minimizing the risk of side effects. Individualization based on patient characteristics, close monitoring, and patient education play vital roles in effective treatment.

CHAPTER SIX

FAQ

What is Simvastatin used for?

Simvastatin is primarily used to lower cholesterol levels, particularly LDL cholesterol, and to reduce the risk of cardiovascular diseases such as heart attacks and strokes. It may also be prescribed for conditions like familial hypercholesterolemia.

How does Simvastatin work?

Simvastatin works by inhibiting the enzyme HMG-CoA reductase, which is involved in cholesterol production in the liver. This leads to decreased levels of LDL cholesterol and triglycerides, and an increase in HDL cholesterol.

What is the usual starting dose of Simvastatin?

The typical starting dose for adults is 10 to 20 mg once daily in the evening. For higher-risk patients, a starting dose of 40 mg may be considered.

Are there any common side effects?

Yes, common side effects of Simvastatin include muscle pain, gastrointestinal issues (such as nausea and diarrhea), headaches, and elevated liver enzymes. Most side effects are mild, but serious effects can occur.

What serious side effects should I be aware of?

Serious side effects include rhabdomyolysis (a severe breakdown of muscle tissue), significant liver damage, and allergic reactions. Symptoms such as severe muscle pain, jaundice, or difficulty breathing should prompt immediate medical attention.

Can I take Simvastatin with other medications?

Simvastatin can interact with various medications, including certain antibiotics, antifungals, and fibrates. It's essential to inform your healthcare provider about all medications and supplements you are taking to avoid potential interactions.

Is there a risk of cognitive effects with Simvastatin?

Some patients have reported memory loss or confusion while taking statins, including Simvastatin. However, evidence on this is mixed. If you experience cognitive changes, discuss them with your healthcare provider.

Can I drink grapefruit juice while taking Simvastatin?

No, grapefruit and grapefruit juice can increase the levels of Simvastatin in your bloodstream, raising the risk of side effects. It's best to avoid grapefruit products while on this medication.

How often should I have my cholesterol checked?

Lipid levels should be checked within 4 to 12 weeks after starting or adjusting the dose of Simvastatin. Follow-up tests can be done every 3 to 12 months, depending on your specific situation.

What should I do if I miss a dose?

If you miss a dose of Simvastatin, take it as soon as you remember. If it's close to the time for your next dose, skip the missed dose and return to your regular schedule. Do not take two doses at once.

Is Simvastatin safe for long-term use?

Simvastatin is considered safe for long-term use in most patients, but regular monitoring is essential to manage potential side effects and ensure optimal cholesterol levels.

Can Simvastatin be taken during pregnancy?

No, Simvastatin is contraindicated during pregnancy due to potential risks to the fetus. Women who are pregnant or planning to become pregnant should discuss alternative treatments with their healthcare provider.

If you have more questions or concerns about Simvastatin, it's always best to consult with your healthcare provider. They can provide personalized information based on your health status and treatment plan.